HMOs
& home remedies
& OTHER JoKes
MEDICAL

LINDA PERRET

cover illustration
DAVID WEBBER MERRELL

inside illustrations
VICKY SNOW

WitWorks™

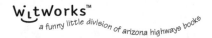

WitWorks™
a funny little division of arizona highways books

2039 West Lewis Avenue, Phoenix, Arizona 85009
Telephone: (602) 712-2200
Web site: www.witworksbooks.com

Publisher — Win Holden
Managing Editor — Bob Albano
Associate Editor — Evelyn Howell
Associate Editor — P. K. McMahon
Art Director — Mary Winkelman Velgos
Photography Director — Peter Ensenberger
Production Director — Cindy Mackey
Production Coordinator — Kim Ensenberger

Library of Congress Catalog Number: 2001097744
ISBN 1-893860-82-5

FIRST EDITION, published in 2002.
Printed in the United States.

Book designer — Mary Winkelman Velgos

When you're not feeling well, you want something – anything – that will cure what ails you. Traditional home remedies fall under the category of *anything*. In this book, under the heading [h o m e   r e m e d y] we list a whole collection of outlandish, bizarre, wacky cure-alls – everything from drinking a concoction of rum and gunpowder to tying a snakeskin around your head. Do they work? Well, I suppose only those who've had courage enough to try them can answer that. We don't recommend that you try them ... not that you would ever want to.

However, they should provide

you with some chuckles, and that's the real purpose of this book. That's why we also included some original lines on hospital life. In here you should find some smiles, a couple of chuckles, maybe some guffaws, and a few belly laughs.

The warning label says, though, "Don't take on a heavy heart."

We believe, and many medical experts agree, that laughter is still the best medicine — and it's cheaper than most prescriptions.

Enjoy and stay well.

— *Linda Perret*

My HMO insurance plan

is a little cheap.

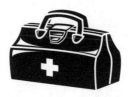

Instead of an anesthesia,

they just provide you

with a flock

of numbered sheep.

To cure a sore throat,
drink hot rum
spiked with gun powder.

Of course it

cures your sore

throat — it

shoots your

tonsils right off.

THE ADMISSIONS CLERK
ASKED ME IF I HAD A
GOOD INSURANCE PLAN.

I SAID,

"OF COURSE.

MY PLAN IS TO

SOMEDAY

BUY SOME."

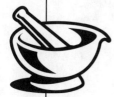

To cure asthma, swallow a handful of spider webs rolled into a ball.

It eases the asthma, but you may be coughing up flies for the next few days.

My doctor firmly believes

in an HMO.

Not the Health Maintenance

Organization kind,

but rather the

Hand Money Over type.

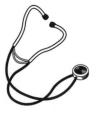

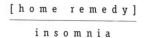

A remedy for insomnia:
Before going to bed, place your feet
in the refrigerator for 10 minutes.

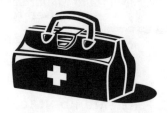

If you are going to try this, it
might be a good idea to put
a couple of Odor-Eaters in the
vegetable crisper.

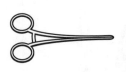 My doctor promised to add 10 years to my life.

HE SAID I'D NEED
THE EXTRA EARNING TIME
TO PAY HIS BILL.

To relieve heartburn,

mix two iceberg lettuce leaves

with six ounces of cold water.

Mash the mixture into a puree

and then drink it slowly.

This remedy is known as
a Salad Shake.

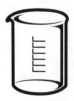

Medicine has changed.

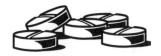

Before it was,

"Take two aspirins and call me in

the morning."

Now it's,

"Take two aspirins and if you

haven't gotten the childproof cap off

by morning, call my service."

Snail broth
was a
remedy for consumption.

"Snail broth" and
"consumption" are
two items I never thought
would ever go together.

MILLIONS OF PEOPLE

BELONG TO HMOs.

I KNOW THIS IS TRUE,

BECAUSE EVERY TIME I

TRY TO SEE MY DOCTOR,

9,999,999

OF 'EM ARE WAITING

AHEAD OF ME.

TO RELIEVE SORE FEET,

HEAT A POT OF BARLEY

UNTIL IT'S THICK.

TAKE OFF THE STOVE AND

WHEN IT IS COOL, PLACE

YOUR FEET IN THE MIXTURE.

When you're done, toss the
stuff. This is one pot of gruel
that even Oliver wouldn't
want more of.

Doctors are always
running tests.

You kind of get the feeling

they are really frustrated

teachers who get paid really,

really well.

One way of

avoiding illness

was not to pay

the doctor

in full.

This is still
being practiced today
by many HMOs.

Doctors want patients
out of the hospital
as quickly as possible.

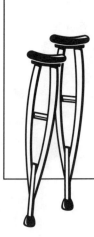

The mechanical
beds
are now
equipped
with an eject
button.

**TO CURE A HEADACHE,
TIE A FLOUR SACK
AROUND YOUR HEAD.**

**All the people
laughing at you
will make you forget
your head
is hurting.**

Your IV contains all your daily

nutrients in one little bag.

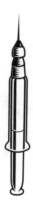

**It would be
downright
perfect if only it
came in
chocolate.**

PIRATES BELIEVED

THAT PIERCING THEIR EARS

AND WEARING EARRINGS

IMPROVED THEIR EYESIGHT.

*If that's true, then
today's punk rockers
should be able to
see in the dark.*

Some people believe HMOs are the best thing to happen to medicine.

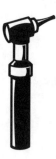

*I think it may be
the same group
that thinks Elvis is alive.*

To cure a fever,
a person would
catch a moth, kill it,
roll it in bacon, and
bury it in the earth.

I'M NOT SURE,

BUT I THINK

THIS WAS

THE BEGINNING OF RUMAKI.

An apple a day

keeps the

doctor away,

but so does

a lousy

healthcare

provider.

To cure bedsores,

place an axe

under your bed.

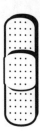

*Just be sure you
know the person
in the bed next to you
really well.*

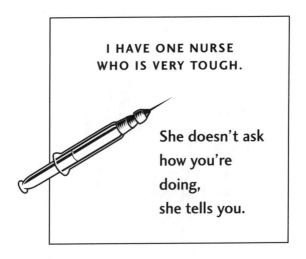

**I HAVE ONE NURSE
WHO IS VERY TOUGH.**

She doesn't ask
how you're
doing,
she tells you.

To cure cramps

in the feet,

turn your shoes

upside down

before going to bed.

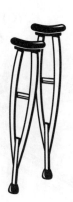

Just be sure to
remove your feet first.

**YOUNG DOCTORS
ARE GOOD.**

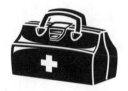

Mine doesn't

charge me as long as

I help him with his

algebra homework.

To eliminate dry mouth,

chew your tongue.

Within half a minute

you should be able

to manufacture

enough saliva

to relieve the dryness.

**If not, just stick out
your tongue
and catch the tears
that will be rolling
down your cheeks.**

NURSES' CORNERS

ARE THE WAY THEY

MAKE THE BEDS WITH

PERFECTLY SQUARE,

VERY TIGHTLY

TUCKED-IN CORNERS.

IT HELPS CUT DOWN

ON ESCAPES.

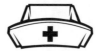

If you have a headache

over one eye,

attach a clothespin

to the lobe of the ear

on the same side

as the pain.

You can cure your headache
and do your laundry
all at the same time.

My doctor is considered
a miracle worker.

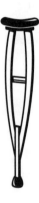 He keeps you sitting

in his waiting room

so long that

whatever you've

got heals itself.

**TO ELIMINATE WARTS,
RUB THEM WITH PEBBLES
AND THROW THEM
INTO A GRAVE.**

The pebbles, not the warts.

**MY MOM AND DAD
WANTED ME TO BE
A DOCTOR.**

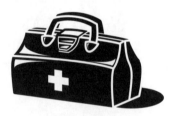

*I think
it was their idea
of long-term
healthcare.*

FOR BURNING FEET,

WRAP TOMATO SLICES

ON THE SOLES OF THE FEET

AND KEEP FEET ELEVATED

FOR HALF AN HOUR.

ADD A COUPLE SLICES OF BACON
AND SOME BREAD, AND NOT ONLY
DO YOU HAVE RELIEF,
BUT ALSO LUNCH.

**I BELONG TO A
HEALTH MAINTENANCE
ORGANIZATION.**

AS LONG AS I

MAINTAIN MY

HEALTH, I CAN BE

PART OF THE

ORGANIZATION.

Throughout history, garlic has been known to improve the voice, the intellect, and the union of broken bones.

But it tends to ruin your social life.

My insurance tries to cut
corners anywhere it can.

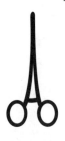

Instead of x-rays,
they just sketch
your insides.

To get rid of ringworm,

mix fountain pen ink

with cigar ashes

and then paint the

affected area with it.

In three to four days,

the ringworm

should be gone.

**LET'S FACE IT. IF YOU PAINTED
ME WITH INK AND ASHES,
I'D SPLIT TOO.**

Doctors have to be a lot of

different things, especially

limber ... that's because

they are constantly bending

over backwards trying to get

the insurance companies

to pay 'em.

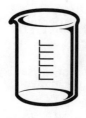 *To stop bleeding, use a mixture of chimney soot and lard.*

IT'S GREASY AND DIRTY,

BUT STILL A LOT BETTER

THAN BLOODY.

**I GUESS I'M
NOT THE BEST PATIENT.**

When it came time to leave,

the nurse didn't wheel me out,

she just opened the window

and tossed me out.

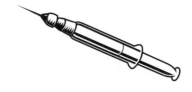

rheumatism

To cure rheumatism,

carry two mole feet

in your breast pocket.

**It also cuts down on
pickpockets.**

MY DOCTOR
WAS SO YOUNG,
HIS BLACK BAG HAD
WINNIE THE POOH
ON IT.

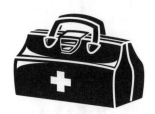

. . . AND A THERMOS IN IT.

TO CURE

SCARLET FEVER,

PATIENTS WERE

DRESSED

ALL IN RED.

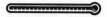

It may not
have helped much,
but they certainly
looked nice.

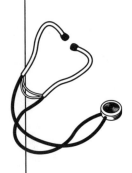

My doctor said
I'd have to give
up alcohol,
tobacco, and
rich expensive
foods for a
month.

Well, he didn't say that;
his bill did.

To cure a sprain,
wrap an eelskin
around it.

Just be sure

it's not

an electric eel;

otherwise a sprain

will be the least

of your worries.

In the hospital,

they give you

three square meals.

I'm gonna use mine

to retile the bathroom.

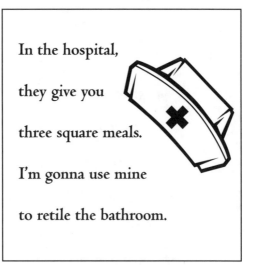

In ancient China,

doctors were prohibited

from seeing their

female patients naked.

Instead, a doll was handed

to the patient, and she would

point to what ailed her.

This process worked well as long as the pain was in her cloth belly, yarn hair, or button eyes.

They have a new procedure
now. Instead of using stitches,
they use a kind of super glue.

Used correctly,
it cuts down on
healing time and scarring.

Used incorrectly,
you spend the rest
of your life with an intern
attached to you.

w o o p i n g   c o u g h

AT ONE TIME,
IT WAS BELIEVED THAT
WHOOPING COUGH
COULD BE CURED
BY GOING TO A BARN
AND INHALING THE
BREATH OF A HORSE.

The only side effect
was a continuous desire
for sugar cubes.

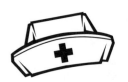 Visitors stop by your room and bring you candy and flowers.

THEY SHOULD BRING

SOMETHING YOU CAN

USE . . . LIKE THE

BOTTOM TO YOUR PAJAMAS.

*To stop sneezing, look at
the tip of your nose
with both eyes.*

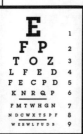

Then pray
your mother
was wrong
and they
don't get
stuck that way.

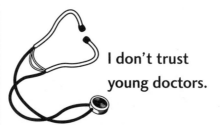

I don't trust
young doctors.

WHEN MY DOCTOR

TELLS ME WHAT TO DO

TO LIVE A LONG LIFE,

I WANT TO KNOW

HE'S SPEAKING

FROM EXPERIENCE.

*To avoid getting the flu,
drink raw sauerkraut juice
every day.*

Between sauerkraut juice

and the flu, I think

I'd prefer the latter.

I wrote a letter to my insurance company complaining about all the paperwork.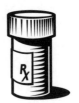

They wrote back — they wanted it in triplicate.

TO CURE INSOMNIA,
CHOP AN ONION AND PUT IT
IN A COVERED JAR. PLACE THE
JAR BESIDE YOUR BED.

IF YOU HAVE TROUBLE
FALLING ASLEEP, OPEN THE
JAR AND TAKE A WHIFF.
COVER THE JAR AGAIN, AND
YOU SHOULD FALL ASLEEP
WITHIN 15 MINUTES.

OF COURSE, YOU MAY DREAM
OF PIZZA, HAMBURGERS,
AND LIVER ALL NIGHT.

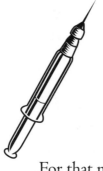

Hospitals can be very expensive. That little IV bottle can cost more than $25 a pop.

For that much, it should

come with an olive

and a little fancy umbrella.

To combat hair loss,

boil one pound of snails

in water.

When the water

has cooled,

wash your hair with it.

*Your hair will still fall out,
but it will be really slow.*

My doctor is very thorough
on his annual physical exams.

ONCE A YEAR

HE DRAWS BLOOD,

MEASURES MY

CHOLESTEROL, TAKES

MY BLOOD PRESSURE,

ROTATES MY TIRES, AND

CHANGES MY OIL.

To get rid of a corn,
rub a candle on a corpse
and then on the corn.

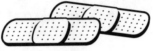

Or just learn to live

with the annoyance

and let the corpse

rest in peace.

Hospital food

is really just

airline meals

that didn't

make the grade.

To reduce varicose veins,
take some cabbage leaves,
and iron them until they
are soft. Place on the
affected areas and hold in
place with bandages. Wear
all day. Repeat daily.

It may not reduce them, but it does make them less noticeable. Let's face it. If you saw a woman walking down the street, what would you notice: the veins on her legs or the nicely pressed cabbage leaves hanging off them?

MY HMO CARES ABOUT ME.

THEY GO THE

EXTRA MILE FOR ME.

I'M MORE THAN JUST

A NUMBER TO THEM.

I KNOW ALL THIS

BECAUSE THEY SENT ME

A LETTER EXPLAINING IT.

IT WAS ADDRESSED,

"DEAR SUBSCRIBER."

To combat fatigue, mix a cup of
water with cayenne pepper and
drink it down.

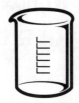

Depending on the strength
of the pepper, this can not
only wake you up but
blow you up, too.

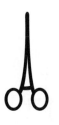 My insurance plan doesn't provide for a private room.

Shoot, I was lucky to get a private bed.

If you wear a pair of red garters

while eating black-eyed peas

with a dime under your plate on

New Year's Day, you will have

health all during the new year.

Of course, you may have to
spend a large portion of it
in the funny farm.

Doctors and nurses

have seen it all,

but a lot of that may

have to do with the

gowns they make you wear.

**To cure
bronchitis,
eat garlic.**

It may not cure you,

but nobody

will get close

enough to you

to find out

you're sick.

NEVER

GO TO A SURGEON

WITH THE NICKNAME

"BUTTERFINGERS."

To reduce the effects of a hangover, rub a quarter of a lemon under each armpit.

This may sound silly,

but it's probably no worse

than what you did

the night before.

Trying to cover yourself
with a hospital gown
is like trying to make
an invitation list
for a wedding.

No matter how hard you try,
someone or something important
is always left out.

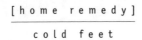

To cure cold feet,

put red pepper pods

in your shoes.

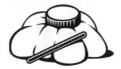

**The other cure is to simply
call off the wedding.**

The experts claim

that HMOs are

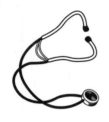

supposed to

bring us quality

medicine at a

reasonable price.

They just forgot to mention
that it was multiple choice.

To cure
a nosebleed,
chew on
a newspaper.

*I don't think I would
want to eat the news.
Just reading it makes me sick.*

I WAS IN THE HOSPITAL

FOR FIVE DAYS.

THREE OF THEM

WERE SPENT

FILLING OUT THE

ADMISSION FORM.

For an ulcer,
cover the soles of your feet
with apple cider vinegar
first thing in the morning,
and again right before dinner.

Worrying about the slop all over your
feet takes your mind off your ulcer.

I don't think I'm the best patient.

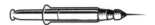

I told the nurse that

the shot in the behind she gave me

didn't make me feel any better.

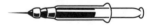

She said, "That's funny.

It worked for me."

**IF SOMEONE IS
TALKING IN HIS SLEEP,
GRAB HIS BIG TOE,
AND THE PERSON WILL
TELL YOU WHATEVER
YOU WANT TO KNOW.**

Most likely,

the only thing

he'll tell you

is to let go

of his toe

I ALWAYS FEEL LIKE

AN ARCHAEOLOGIST

WHEN I'M IN

MY DOCTOR'S

WAITING ROOM.

I never know what I'm going to find,
but chances are, it'll be old.

TO RELIEVE STRESS,
CHOP AN ONION
INTO SMALL BITS AND
ADD A TABLESPOON
OF HONEY.

EAT HALF THE MIXTURE
AT LUNCH AND
THE OTHER HALF
WITH DINNER.

Just knowing
I was going to
have to swallow
this goo would
cause me stress.

There are only two good reasons
for going to the hospital.

One is to have a baby and the
other is to have plastic surgery.

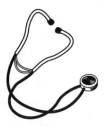

*In both cases, you check out
with a brand-new body.*

To eliminate the problem

of gas pains,

stand on your head.

Stay upside down

for a minute.

This will relieve

the gas, and the only

side effect

is you could possibly

break your neck.

My doctor
said I was a
hypochondriac
and that
my illness
wasn't real.

**I GOT EVEN WITH HIM —
THE CHECK I SENT HIM
ISN'T REAL EITHER.**

To cure mumps,
you should rub your neck
along the front edge
of a hog trough.

THE ONLY REAL SIDE

EFFECT IS YOU DEVELOP

A HIGH-PITCHED SQUEAL

AND YOUR TAIL STARTS

TO CURL UP A BIT.

Hospitals are strange.

THEY TELL YOU

TO KEEP WARM

AND THEN MAKE YOU

WEAR A GOWN

WITH BUILT-IN

AIR CONDITIONING.

s w i m m e r ' s   e a r

For swimmer's ear, fill

an eardropper with vodka and

squeeze a few drops into the ear,

then let it drain out.

Drain it out into
a glass with ice,
add an olive, and
you have a cure and a vodka martini.

HAVING VISITORS
IN THE HOSPITAL IS GREAT.

They're the only people

who stop by your room

and don't send you

a bill later on.

**To ward off all diseases,
hair was taken from the
cross on the back of a donkey
and worn in a charm
around the neck.**

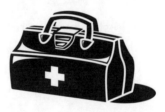

*I think this really got started by a
guy who was too cheap to buy his
girl a diamond necklace.*

*My HMO doesn't view me
as just another number.*

No, I'm more than that.

I'm a premium

that's due on the

first of each month.

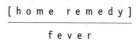

For a fever,
bind sliced onions
to the bottoms
of your feet.

After all, if you're going to feel stinky,
you might as well dress the part.

Medicine
is a vicious cycle.

You feel sick, you go
to the doctor, he
makes you better,
sends you a bill,
and then you feel
sick again.

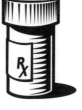

To keep from

getting a headache,

tie a snake skin

around your head.

It may keep

your headache away,

but it tends to

tick off the snake.

GOOD BEDSIDE MANNERS.

THAT'S A DOCTOR WHO

CAN STIFLE A LAUGH WHEN

HE SEES YOU NAKED.

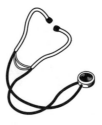

For coughing,

make a syrup of kerosene oil

mixed with molasses and

a dash of turpentine.

It stops your coughing, but also
stops your breathing.

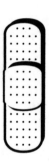 Hospitals can work miracles. They can turn an ordinary Band-Aid into a $6.75 item on your bill.

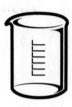

Chicken soup was a remedy for constipation.

Although, it didn't seem to help the chicken.

THE WAY THEY KEEP

PUSHING JELL-O

ON YOU, YOU'D

THINK THE

HEAD NURSE WAS

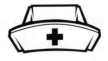

BILL COSBY.

To stop bleeding,
place a spider web
across the wound.

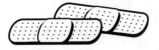

IT NOT ONLY

STOPS THE

BLEEDING,

BUT ALSO IS A

HANDY WAY TO

CATCH INSECTS.

**THERE ARE CERTAIN TOOLS
OF THE TRADE A GOOD
DOCTOR NEEDS.**

A stethoscope,

a thermometer,

tongue depressors,

and a nurse who knows

where all of them

are kept.

sore throat

To cure a sore throat,
wear one of your
long stockings
around your neck
with the foot
under your chin.

To avoid other discomforts,
be sure the sock is clean.

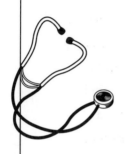

**My doctor told
me I would have
to start eating
right.**

I would have believed her, too,
if she hadn't been chomping
on a Milky Way at the time.

In ancient China,

doctors were paid

when their patients

were kept well,

not when they were sick.

If a patient got

sick too often,

the doctor had to

pay the patient.

Some things should

never change.

Second opinion:

That's the medical way

of saying,

"Hey, don't blame me."

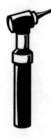 To cure catarrh,
snuff lemon juice
mixed with honey
up your nose
four times a day.

**THIS JUST DOESN'T
MAKE SENSE.**

**YOUR NOSTRILS
WILL PUCKER FROM
THE LEMON JUICE
AND STICK THAT WAY
FROM THE HONEY.**

I PLAY GOLF WITH MY
DOCTOR, BUT HE MAKES ME
KEEP SCORE.

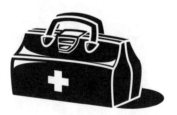

HE SAYS HE HAS ENOUGH
PAPER WORK AT THE OFFICE.

To cure arthritis, drink a mixture of honey, vinegar, and whiskey.

*If you put in enough of the last ingredient, you can cure **all** your aches and pains.*

If you are trying

to get your bills paid,

it doesn't matter

if you belong to

an H-M-O or a P-P-O,

their answer will still

be the same . . .

N-O.

For a bad back it was recommended that you heat cabbage leaves, massage a little olive oil into the painful area, place the cabbage over the oil, and wrap in a hot towel.

ADD A LITTLE CORN BEEF,

AND THIS REMEDY BECOMES

VERY POPULAR AROUND THE

17TH OF MARCH.

It's okay
that doctors make
lots of money . . .

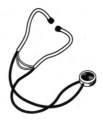

would you trust
your kidneys to someone
who drove a '78 Pinto?

For a cramp,

a ring made

from the handle

of a decayed coffin

was to be worn

on the finger all night.

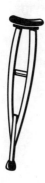

*Of course, poking
around a cemetery
looking for
decayed coffins
was probably what
caused the cramp
in the first place.*

My doctor is very
friendly . . . at least
that's what the
nurses keep saying.

*To cure a child
from whooping cough,
it was recommended
that a trout's head be placed
in the child's mouth.*

Of course,

the kid has to spend

the rest of his life

with the nickname

"Fishface."

I had a very tough nurse

while I was in the hospital.

It's the first time I've ever seen

a billy club used as a

medical instrument.

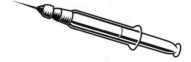

May dew was used as a lotion for
improving the complexion.

You just had to be
careful where the
dew came from.

**IT WOULD BE TERRIBLE TO
HAVE SMOOTH SKIN COVERED
IN CRABGRASS.**

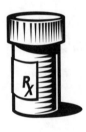 I'm not real confident about my doctor. He got an "A" in penmanship.

To ward off toothaches,

measles, and other

childhood diseases,

a person was to ride

a donkey facing its tail.

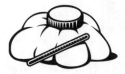

*Although it didn't do much
to eliminate the pain from
riding into a brick wall.*

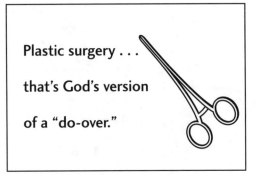

Plastic surgery . . .

that's God's version

of a "do-over."

A cure for asthma
was to drink tea made
from the bark of a wild plum.

Your asthma
would be gone,
but you might
end up with a
terrible case of
root rot.

**I LOVE TO VISIT THE NURSERY
AT THE HOSPITAL.**

I look through the glass window

and see our hope for tomorrow

wrapped up like tiny burritos.

To cure chest congestion,

boil a cup of white wine

and carefully

inhale the vapor.

Avoid driving after this

procedure, as this could be a

little tricky explaining if you

got pulled over.

Doctor's orders:

That's the adult version

of Simon Says.

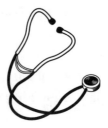

*To get rid of a sty
on your eyelid, rub your
grandmother's wedding ring
across it nine times.*

*Unless your grandfather
was really cheap.*

*In that case, not only would
you still have the sty, but your
eyelid would turn green.*

I THINK MY KIDS

ARE GOING TO GROW UP

TO BE DOCTORS.

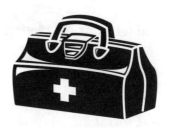

**WHEN I CALL THEM,
THEY NEVER RESPOND.**

If you want your mustache

to grow, put sweet milk or

cream on your

lip and let

a cat lick it off.

It's not recommended that
women try this one.

Hospitals are strange.

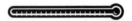

THE DOCTORS

KEEP MAKING YOU WELL,

WHILE THE CHEF

KEEPS MAKING YOU SICK.

Since ancient times,

garlic has been used

to cure intestinal worms.

It not only gets rid of the worms,
but also keeps vampires away.

A hospital gown . . .

the true meaning

of southern exposure.

TO CURE A CHILD OF ASTHMA,
BORE A HOLE INTO A DOORJAMB
JUST LEVEL WITH THE HEAD OF
THE CHILD.

PLACE ONE HAIR FROM THE
CHILD INTO THE HOLE, AND
COVER WITH PUTTY.

WHEN THE CHILD GROWS
TALLER THAN THE HOLE,
HE WILL BE CURED.

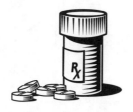

*But the value of your home
will have dipped slightly.*

A nurse said to me, "Do you know the difference between a biscuit and a plaster cast?

I said, "No."

She said, "Then you're going to love lunch."

To cure asthma,

hold

a Chihuahua.

Your asthma will

transfer

to the dog.

This remedy may work, but it puts an end to the "man's best friend" thing.

MY DOCTOR

IS KIND OF

OLD-FASHIONED.

HIS FAVORITE

PROCEDURE IS

LEECHING.

For feverish
chills, it was
recommended
that the patient
walk over the
boundaries of
nine fields in
one day.

Of course, then
you'd have to
look up the
remedy for
sore feet.

I made an astounding
discovery while
in the hospital.

**EVERYONE I KNOW
IS A LIAR.**

They all walked in the
room and said,
"You look great."

To cure "gucky" eyes,

it was recommended that

you dip cotton balls in egg white

and place over your eyes.

Bind them in place

and go to sleep.

In the morning, your eyes

should be clear.

**PROVIDED, OF COURSE,
YOU REMEMBER TO
REMOVE THE COTTON BALLS.**

Nowadays,
doctors
all have
fancy titles.

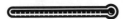

**THE OTHER DAY
I WENT TO A
QUACKOLOGIST.**

**To fight off nausea,
peel a large onion,
cut it in half, and place
one half under each armpit.**

*Apparently, it's very hard
to be sick while holding onions
with your armpits.*

*In fact, it's pretty hard to do
just about anything
while holding onions
with your armpits.*

When you check out of the hospital, they hand you a plastic bag with all your possessions.

IT'S NOT A COURTESY. THAT'S ALL YOU'VE GOT LEFT AFTER PAYING THE BILL.

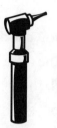

To ease a stuffy nose,

rub your ears vigorously

until they feel as if

they are burning.

THIS SHOULD CLEAR UP

THE STUFFY NOSE,

BUT YOUR HAIR

MAY CATCH FIRE.

I had a
tough RN
in the hospital.
She had a blackbelt
in nursing.

[home remedy]

jaundice

*To cure jaundice,
the skin of a lizard was placed
under the patient's pillow.*

FINDING OUT

THEY SLEPT WITH

THE REMAINS OF A LIZARD

WOULD MAKE MOST PEOPLE

TURN WHITE.